The Power of Intermittent Fasting
Transform Your Health and Waistline

Table of Contents

Chapter 1. Introduction

Indulge yourself in our Special Report, 'The Power of Intermittent Fasting: Transform Your Health and Waistline.' This guide is much more than a dietary plan—it's your key to unlock an invigorating lifestyle transformation! Through the simple power of intermittent fasting, you'll discover profound insights into improving your health, waistline, and overall vitality. Strikingly straightforward and filled with illuminating research, this report unpacks the wonders of intermittent fasting's influence on your well-being in a way that fits smoothly into your daily life. Lastly, it cultivates a constructive mindset, paving the way to a healthier you. So don't wait around! This report is the catalyst for the magnificent change you're seeking for your health and body shape. Take a minute and bag your copy. Remember, the journey to a transformed you begins only with a choice!

Chapter 2. Understanding Intermittent Fasting

Intermittent fasting is not merely a dietary fad that's currently taking the wellness world by storm—it's a practice that has been around for centuries, one that our ancestors unknowingly depended on. Modern research now points out the various ways this simple lifestyle adjustment can significantly impact our health and wellness, which has led to its soaring popularity.

The principle of intermittent fasting is surprisingly simple: cycle between periods of eating and fasting. However, the magic lies not in the simplicity of its principle but in the profoundity of its effects.

2.1. Discerning Various Intermittent Fasting Protocols

Intermittent Fasting (IF) comes in various forms, each with its unique balances of eating and fasting windows. The following are the most popular IF protocols:

1. 16/8 method: This involves daily fasts of 16 hours for men and 14-15 hours for women. Eating windows range from 8-10 hours. It is often called the 'Leangains protocol,' popularized by fitness expert Martin Berkhan.

2. 5:2 diet: This demands two days of reduced calorie intake (around 500-600 calories) every week. Practitioners eat normally on the remaining five days, often termed 'fast' and 'feed' days respectively.

3. Eat-Stop-Eat: This method involves 24-hour fasting, once or twice a week, with normal eating on other days.

4. Warrior Diet: This is a daylong fast followed by a large meal at

night, mimicking the dietary practices of ancient warriors.

The choice of protocol varies depending on individual health conditions, weight-loss goals, lifestyles, and comfort. Each approach has its merits, so take the time to choose what suits you best.

2.2. The Biological Clock and Intermittent Fasting

The human body is designed to function on a specific timetable set by our biological clocks, or circadian rhythms. Circadian rhythms are essentially 24-hour cycles that regulate our bodily functions, including sleep, appetite, hormone release, and cell regeneration, among many.

This rhythm dictates how our bodies metabolize food, influencing our weight, energy levels, and overall health. Unfortunately, with the advent of artificial lighting, extended working hours, and faulty eating habits, our circadian rhythm is often disrupted, opening doors to various health problems. When we practice intermittent fasting, we essentially reset our biological clock, allowing it to function as it should—leading us to sustain optimal levels of health.

2.3. The Science Behind Fasting

During the fasting state, you're not providing your body with caloric energy. As a result, your body shifts its source of fuel from the glucose derived from your most recent meal to the stored glycogen in your muscles and liver. Eventually, as these stores deplete, your body turns to stored fat.

When fat is metabolically processed, free fatty acids get converted into ketone bodies, or ketones, in your liver. These ketones are used as energy by your brain and body in the absence of glucose. This is why fasting aids in weight loss—it's a metabolic switch from using glucose as a primary energy source to using fats.

During prolonged fasting, insulin decreases, and human growth hormone (HGH) levels increase. The elevated HGH enables fat burning and muscle gain while lowering insulin, further driving your body to use stored fat for fuel.

2.4. Fasting and Autophagy

Autophagy, derived from the Greek words 'auto' (self) and 'phagy' (eat), is a cellular "cleaning out" process that occurs during fasting. As the body's way of conducting spring cleaning, autophagy breaks down and recycles damaged parts of cells like misfolded proteins, which, if left unrepaired, can lead to various diseases such as cancer, Alzheimer's, and infections.

Fasting triggers autophagy, thereby helping the body detoxify, repair, and rejuvenate on a cellular level. This has a wholesome effect on overall health and longevity.

2.5. Intermittent Fasting and Mental Health

Many practitioners of intermittent fasting report increased mental clarity and concentration during the fasting period. It is believed to be due to the cognitive enhancement effects of ketones.

In addition to this, fasting also stimulates the production of Brain-Derived Neurotrophic Factor (BDNF), a protein that supports cognitive function by encouraging the survival of existing neurons and growth of new neurons.

Better mental performance, with an increased sense of well-being, further fuel the practice of intermittent fasting for optimum health.

Understanding intermittent fasting is the first step toward revolutionizing your health and lifestyle. By adopting a pattern of cyclical fasting, you invite a host of benefits from weight loss and increased energy levels, to enhanced mental clarity, decreased inflammation, and elevated overall vitality. So why wait? Start your journey today.

Chapter 3. The Science Behind Intermittent Fasting

The transformative power of intermittent fasting (IF), a pattern of eating that cycles eating and fasting, is founded in science. Our ancestors, who were hunter-gatherers, followed a similar eating pattern as they didn't have a stable food supply. This lifestyle compelled our bodies to adapt and perform optimally even without frequent meals. Today, our bodies still retain this metabolic flexibility, making intermittent fasting a viable option not only for weight control but also for improved overall health.

3.1. Origin and Evolution

IF is far from being a modern invention. Our ancestors unknowingly deployed it thousands of years ago, given their unpredictable access to food. It was only much later that humans came to associate the timetable of the sun with the schedule of eating, therefore tying it to the circadian rhythm. Modern lifestyles have disrupted this balance, with constant access to food and deviation from natural light and dark cycles. These disruptions have contributed to the characteristic disease patterns we witness today, such as obesity and diabetes.

3.2. The Fasting State: A Closer Look

Let's delve into what happens within your body during fasting. Approximately eight hours after your last meal, your body enters a state of fasting. When you consume a meal, the body utilizes glucose as its primary form of energy and stores the surplus as glycogen in your liver and muscles. During a fast, as the kidneys reabsorb glucose and insulin levels drop, the body needs to use its stored glycogen for energy. Once the glycogen stores are exhausted, usually around 10-12 hours into the fast, your body starts burning stored fat for energy. This metabolic transition is known as 'ketosis'. Your body also induces a process called 'autophagy', essentially a cellular clean-up, that recycles cells and proteins that have outlived their usefulness.

3.3. Intermittent Fasting and Metabolic Health

Intermittent fasting can significantly improve health-related outcomes. Many studies have shown that IF can modify diverse aspects of health, such as insulin resistance, cardiovascular health, neurodegenerative diseases, and cancer.

It's essential to understand that insulin resistance, a significant driver of many chronic diseases like diabetes, obesity, heart disease, and many cancers, can be effectively managed with intermittent fasting. When you fast, insulin levels drop and human growth hormone increases. Your cells also change the expression of genes, which helps resistance against disease.

3.4. Interplay with Circadian Rhythm

Robust research suggests that aligning our eating patterns to our natural circadian rhythm (the built-in 24-hour biological clock governing our sleep-wake cycle) is beneficial. The alignment fundamentally improves digestion, lets each system in your body prepare for nutrient absorption, metabolism, and repair, and also optimizes body weight and composition. IF can be a helpful tool in restoring our natural circadian rhythm, disrupted by late-night screen time, sleep disturbances, and irregular meal times.

3.5. Hormonal Changes and Weight Loss

The most evident upshot of IF, one that also serves as its most substantial paradigm of appeal, is weight loss. The biological mechanisms for this are anchored in the hormonal changes that occur during a fasting state. IF significantly lowers insulin levels, allowing fat cells to release their stored energy to be used up. It also leads to a significant rise in the human growth hormone, which facilitates fat burning and muscle gain.

Moreover, fasting induces changes in the function of hormones, genes, and cells that are related to longevity and protection against disease. For instance, IF enhances the body's resistance to oxidative stress, reducing tissue damage and preventing aging and the onset of diverse diseases.

3.6. Findings from Human and Animal Studies

Scientific literature flourishes with both human and animal studies endorsing IF's effects on health and longevity. Studies on rats have shown increased lifespan, improved health, and slowed disease progression when subjected to intermittent fasting. Similarly, observational studies with fasting humans have noted improvements in markers like blood pressure, LDL and total cholesterol, insulin resistance, and body weight.

3.7. The Big Picture: Intermittent Fasting and Longevity

Many researches argue that both the metabolic and hormonal changes triggered by IF can facilitate an increased lifespan. These changes, including lower insulin and sugar levels, increased human growth hormone, enhanced cellular repair processes, and altered gene expressions, not only support healthy aging but also offer resistance against several diseases.

In conclusion, intermittent fasting is a powerful, scientifically-backed adjustment to our eating habits that can bring about remarkable health benefits. It roots in our ancestral heritage and works well with our biological inclinations, favoring a minimalist, naturalistic approach to eating that does away with the complications of calorie counting or restrictive dieting.

Through intermittent fasting, we can harness the inherent adaptability of our bodies, optimize our health and longevity, and build a concrete foundation towards a transformative lifestyle change. As with any significant lifestyle alteration, it's recommended to incorporate and adhere to it guided by professional healthcare advice, tuned to your specific health requirements and body profile.

Chapter 4. Different Approaches to Intermittent Fasting

Intermittent fasting (IF) is a dietary approach that revolves around periods of eating and fasting. The aim is not to dictate what foods you should eat but rather when you should eat them. There isn't one definitive method for intermittent fasting; it can be adapted based on individual lifestyles and eating preferences. Below we delve into the most popular methods, shedding light on the schedules, benefits, and challenges of each.

4.1. The 16/8 Method

Arguably the most popular type of intermittent fasting, the 16/8 method is characterized by eating within an 8-hour window and fasting for the remaining 16 hours of the day. It's also known as the Leangains protocol.

Typically, the fasting period includes the time you spend sleeping. To practice this method, you can merely skip breakfast and make lunch your first meal of the day. Some people, however, prefer to eat between 9 a.m. and 5 p.m., while others start their eating window later.

This method is lauded for its flexibility and ease of incorporation into daily life. Besides, the 16/8 method is conducive to maintaining muscle mass while concurrently aiding in weight loss, particularly if combined with resistance training.

4.2. The 5:2 Diet

The 5:2 diet, or the 'Fast Diet,' involves eating normally for five days of the week and restricting your calorie intake to 500–600 calories for the remaining two non-consecutive days. On the two fasting days, it is often recommended that women consume 500 calories and men 600 calorie.

A typical week might involve normal eating from Monday to Friday, with restricted calorie intake on Saturday and Sunday. It could also involve inserting the fasting days amidst the traditional eating days. This method, popularized by British journalist Michael Mosley, is especially appealing due to its simplicity and the fact that it doesn't require total fasting.

4.3. Eat Stop Eat

This approach necessitates a 24-hour fast once or twice a week. The Eat Stop Eat method, advocated by fitness expert Brad Pilon, requires that you eat normally for five to six days of the week and fast completely—unlike the 5:2 method—for one to two days.

During the fasting days, no food is allowed, although you can drink calorie-free beverages. Once the fasting period is over, you can return to your regular eating habits. Keep in mind, though, it's essential not to compensate for the fasting days by overeating on non-fasting days.

4.4. Alternate Day Fasting

With alternate day fasting, you subject yourself to full 24-hour fasting periods every other day. On some versions of this diet, you are allowed 500 calories on fasting days. However, total fasting makes this method more extreme than others.

This diet's effectivity is currently a subject of ongoing research, though preliminary data indicates that alternate day fasting could lead to significant health improvements.

4.5. Spontaneous Meal Skipping

This method involves skipping meals when convenient. If you're not hungry, too busy, or simply don't feel like eating—just don't. This type of IF emphasizes listening to your body, eating when hungry, and not eating out of habit or due to social cues.

While spontaneous meal skipping may not be as structured as other IF methods, it encourages intuitive eating, making it a more sustainable long-term practice to most.

4.6. Warrior Diet

The Warrior Diet, created by fitness author Ori Hofmekler, involves eating small amounts of raw fruits and vegetables during the day and one big meal at night—your 'feast.' Essentially, you fast all day—20 hours—then overeat in a 4-hour evening window.

This diet, based on the eating patterns of ancient warriors who consumed little during the day and feasted at night, is lauded for its focus on whole, unprocessed foods. It also allows for increased food enjoyment and satisfaction during the feasting window.

Intermittent fasting isn't a one-size-fits-all concept. You have the flexibility to choose a method that suits your lifestyle and health needs. Before embarking on any IF routine, it's always wise to consult with a healthcare provider, especially if you have any existing health conditions. Just remember: no matter the method, intermittent fasting should encourage a healthier relationship with food, not a restrictive one. It's a tool for wellness, not a punishment.

Chapter 5. Potential Health Benefits of Intermittent Fasting

Intermittent fasting has recently been hailed as a new health panacea with impressive potential for dealing with a wide range of health issues. It is often described as a dietary rhythm that alternates between periods of eating and fasting. This method of structureed eating not only prompts weight loss but also improves metabolic health and even extends the lifespan in animals.

5.1. How Intermittent Fasting Works

To understand the potential health benefits of intermittent fasting, we must first understand how it works. When we eat, our body spends a few hours processing that food, burning what it can from what we've just consumed. Because it is more convenient to burn food as energy than it is to burn stored fat, our bodies turn to the energy readily available from our recent meal.

However, during fasting states, your body doesn't have a recently consumed meal to use as energy, so it is more likely to pull from the fat stored in your body, rather than from glucose in your blood stream or glycogen in your muscles/liver. In this sense, intermittent fasting allows our bodies to use their stored energy.

5.2. Weight Loss and Intermittent Fasting

One of the most impactful benefits of intermittent fasting is its potential for weight loss. Regular implementation of some fasting modes can enhance the body's responsiveness to insulin, helping to manage weight and reduce the risk of obesity-related diseases such as type 2 diabetes and heart disease.

During fasting periods, the body will try to conserve energy by reducing the amount of unnecessary energy expenditure, which can lead to weight loss. Additionally, when in a fasted state, the body routes blood to different parts of the body, such as to the muscles for repair and growth, which can result in lean body mass increase while fat mass decreases.

5.3. Healthier Heart

Scientists have long known about the link between eating patterns and heart health. Today's typical pattern of continuous eating interspersed with snacking may contribute to the high levels of heart disease and stroke. However, emerging research has shown that intermittent fasting can lead to reductions in blood pressure, cholesterol levels, and heart rate, all of which are significant factors in maintaining a healthier heart.

In this sense, intermittent fasting helps to ensure that heart cells work efficiently, are healthy, and can regenerate after damage. Furthermore, it has a positive impact on factors that directly influence heart health including blood pressure, cholesterol levels, and levels of inflammatory markers.

5.4. Neurological Health and Intermittent Fasting

In addition to physical health benefits, intermittent fasting can enhance mental acuity and has been linked with protecting against neurodegenerative diseases. Evidence from animal studies has suggested that this dietary habit can improve brain function, possibly increasing the growth of new neurons and protecting the brain from damage.

Additionally, levels of a brain hormone called brain-derived neurotrophic factor (BDNF) may increase. This could have protective effects against depression and other mental health disorders. Furthermore, a dietary pattern like intermittent fasting could help to reduce inflammation, often considered a primary cause in chronic conditions such as Parkinson's and Alzheimer's diseases.

5.5. Autophagy: The Cellular Cleaning Process

Autophagy, which translates to "self-eating," is a cellular cleaning process that happens more prominently when we fast. This process involves the body's cells breaking down and metabolizing broken and dysfunctional proteins that build up inside cells over time.

Increased autophagy can have numerous health benefits. From a cellular perspective, it helps to reduce inflammation and bolster the immune system. On a wider level, it could enhance general health and longevity. Evidence suggests that intermittent fasting can increase the rate of autophagy, helping to promote cellular health and functionality, which might guard against various diseases, including cancer and heart disease.

5.6. Enhanced Physical Performance

Intermittent fasting can also have benefits relating to physical performance. When implemented correctly, it can induce physiological adaptations that enhance stamina and fitness. After a period of adjustment, most individuals report increased energy levels and improved physical performance during fasts. Research is ongoing, but initial observations suggest that endurance and resistance training responses could be optimized through a well-managed fasting regimen, which might be of interest to athletes and fitness enthusiasts.

In conclusion, while the research into intermittent fasting is still emerging, it is increasingly clear that it could offer significant advantages for many individuals. Those looking to enhance their general health, lose weight, or simply seek a new and refreshing approach to their diet might consider the potential benefits of intermittent fasting. However, as with any diet plan, the guidance of a healthcare provider is essential to ensure safety and efficacy.

Chapter 6. Intermittent Fasting and Weight Loss

When it comes to weight loss, one must understand a core principle at the heart of it all: to lose weight, you must burn more calories than you consume. This can be achieved in two ways: by reducing your caloric intake or increasing the amount of calories burned through physical activities. Here's where intermittent fasting comes into play—it significantly helps in limiting caloric intake over a specific period.

6.1. Understanding the Basics of Intermittent Fasting

Intermittent fasting is not just another fad diet—it's a lifestyle choice that involves eating within a specific time frame during the day and fasting for the remaining time. This defined pattern of eating and refraining does not specify what foods to eat; instead, it focuses on when to eat.

There are several methods of intermittent fasting, primarily differing in the duration of the eating and fasting periods. The 16/8 method, for instance, involves restraining from eating for 16 hours and limiting all consumption to an 8-hour window. Other popular methods are the eat-stop-eat method, which involves fasting for 24 hours once or twice a week, and the 5:2 diet, in which individuals limit their calorie intake to 500–600 on two nonconsecutive days of the week and eat normally on the other five days.

6.2. The Science Behind Intermittent Fasting and Weight Loss

Research shows a significant correlation between intermittent fasting and weight loss. How does it work? Well, the critical factor here is the body's shifting metabolic state during the fasting and eating periods.

When we eat, especially carbohydrates, our body converts these foods into glucose, which our cells use for energy. Excess glucose is stored as glycogen in the liver. But our liver can store only a limited amount of glycogen. When we continue to consume more than required, the excess accumulates as fat.

When we stop eating for a prolonged period due to fasting, our glycogen stores deplete—we've used all the readily available fuel. As a result, our body switches its fuel source from glycogen to fat, thus entering a state of ketosis. This switch to burning fat as a primary source of energy significantly aids weight loss.

In addition to encouraging weight loss, intermittent fasting has been linked to several other health benefits. These include reduced inflammation, improved heart health and insulin sensitivity, enhanced brain function, and increased life longevity.

6.3. Practical Ways to Incorporate Intermittent Fasting in your Lifestyle

Successfully following an intermittent fasting lifestyle requires strategic planning. It's not just about skipping meals; there are important considerations to take into account to maximize the benefits and minimize potential issues.

First, you need to choose an intermittent fasting method that fits into your lifestyle. For example, if you're a breakfast person, the 16/8 method—where you skip the evening meal—might be suitable for you. On the other hand, if dinner is your most substantial meal, you might want to skip breakfast instead.

Second, during your eating windows, ensure you consume a balance of nutrients. It's essential to maintain adequate protein intake and include plenty of fruits, vegetables, whole grains, and healthy fats in your diet. This nutrient-dense approach will keep you feeling satisfied and provide the necessary vitamins and minerals for overall health.

Third, listen to your body. If you're feeling unwell or weak, it might be a good idea to ease into the practice slowly. Starting with shorter fasting periods and gradually increasing the duration can help in this adaptation process.

Always remember, it's crucial to stay hydrated during the fasting periods. During your fast, you can drink water, coffee, and other non-caloric beverages to curb hunger pangs. If you keep yourself hydrated, you are less likely to feel hungry, and also it helps to keep your body functions moving smoothly.

6.4. Overcoming Challenges in Intermittent Fasting

Embarking on an intermittent fasting journey isn't without challenges. Common obstacles include cravings, overeating in eating periods, lack of social understanding, low energy, or difficulties adjusting to the new lifestyle.

To overcome these challenges, it's essential to plan. Have a list of healthy meals ready for your eating windows to avoid succumbing to cravings. Aim to eat until you're satisfied, not stuffed. Inform your social circle about your fasting lifestyle so they can support your journey.

In summary, intermittent fasting is a promising weight-loss strategy that also offers additional health benefits. It is flexible and can be tailored to fit various lifestyles and dietary preferences. In conjunction with a balanced diet and regular physical activity, intermittent fasting can indeed be a powerful tool in reaching your health and weight loss goals.

Chapter 7. Strategies for Successful Intermittent Fasting

Success with intermittent fasting is not just about what and when you eat. It's a lifestyle change that requires strategic planning and considered execution. In this chapter, we'll go deep into the strategies that can help you succeed in your intermittent fasting journey, examining everything from mental preparation, meal planning, fitness, and hydration, to managing hunger pangs and dealing with social events.

7.1. Mental Preparation

Before you embark on your intermittent fast, it's paramount to prepare mentally. Understand that it's not a diet but a lifestyle. Facing challenges is part of the journey, and having a strong willpower can make a significant difference in your fasting journey.

1. Determine Your Goals: Define what you aim to achieve with intermittent fasting. It could be for better health, weight loss, or improved cognitive function.

2. Set Realistic Expectations: Instant gratification is unrealistic. Intermittent fasting requires patience and commitment. Weight loss and health improvement occur gradually.

3. Prepare For Hunger: Being mentally prepared for hunger is an essential part of the journey. It may feel intense initially, but your body will gradually adapt.

7.2. Meal Planning

Meal planning can help to maximize the benefits of fasting periods. Here's how you can develop an effective meal plan:

1. Eat Balanced Meals: Your meals should include an ample amount of proteins, healthy fats, and low-GI carbohydrates.

2. Time Your Carbohydrate Intake: Eating most of your carbs after your workout can enhance glycogen storage and muscle repair.

3. Stay Hydrated: Hydration is critical. Be sure to hydrate regularly throughout the day, especially during fasting hours.

4. Supplements: Consider taking vitamins and supplements to ensure you receive the right nutrients during your feeding window.

7.3. Fitness and Intermittent Fasting

Fasting and exercise are symbiotic: they both enhance the effects of the other when done correctly.

1. Adjust Your Workout Schedule: During the adaptation period, schedule your workouts near the end of your fasting window and eat your first meal afterward.

2. Listen To Your Body: If you feel too tired, it might be a sign that you're pushing too hard. Adjust your intensity as needed.

7.4. Managing Hunger Pangs

Initially, hunger pangs can be a challenge. However, with time and a few tricks, you can manage it effectively.

1. Stay Busy: Boredom can lead to thoughts of eating. Filling your day with engaging activities will help distract from hunger pangs.

2. Green Tea: A cup of green tea during your fasting window will not only provide anti-oxidants but also has appetite-curbing properties.

3. Carbonated Water: Carbonated water can give a feeling of fullness, helping curb the urge to eat.

7.5. Social Commitments

Social situations where food is involved can pose a challenge while fasting.

1. Make a Plan: If you know you have a social commitment, adjust your eating schedule for the day to accommodate the event.

2. Eat Ahead of Time: If you can't adjust your fasting window, consider having a small meal before your event.

Remember, intermittent fasting's goal is to improve your health and quality of life. It should never be a source of stress. Be flexible and make intermittent fasting adapt to your lifestyle, not the other way around. After all, consistency is key, and adopting these strategies will ensure your success on your journey to better health and a slimmer waistline.

Chapter 8. Overcoming Common Challenges in Intermittent Fasting

Intermittent fasting is an eating habit that entails specifying periods of feeding and fasting. While compelling research points to its numerous health benefits, it does pose some challenges, especially for beginners. These trials range from physiological to psychological, and even social issues. However, they are manageable, and with the appropriate techniques and mindset, you can successfully transition into and sustain an intermittent fasting lifestyle.

8.1. Understanding Hunger and Cravings

Hunger is the main challenge confronting beginners in intermittent fasting. It's natural to feel hungry when you commence fasting; however, it's vital to discern actual hunger from food cravings. Our bodies communicate the need for vital nutrients through hunger—a physical need, distinct from cravings that are emotionally driven desires mostly towards specific types of food. Understanding this difference can help you manage your feeding periods efficiently and quell unnecessary snacking that could limit the benefits of your fast.

To mitigate hunger, ensure your meals incorporate enough protein, healthy fats, and fiber. These macronutrients promote a feeling of satiety, reducing your cravings. Additionally, consistently consuming water, herbal tea, or black coffee during the fasting period can help alleviate hunger.

8.2. Dealing with Fatigue

As you transition into intermittent fasting, you might experience fatigue. This tiredness results from your body adjusting to the new eating schedule and burning stored fats for energy, a process known as ketosis. While this is a typical response, it's critical to monitor your body to ensure it's not due to underlying conditions, or severe calorie restriction, both of which require medical intervention.

To counteract fatigue, ensure your diet includes nutrient-dense foods, particularly those rich in iron, such as spinach and other leafy greens, and proteins. Hydrating adequately also helps as dehydration often manifests in the form of fatigue. Moderate exercise can increase energy levels and contribute to positive well-being.

8.3. Maintaining Nutritional Adequacy

Generally, intermittent fasting doesn't dictate what to eat but when to eat. Consequently, it's possible to fall into a trap of inadequate diet quality if your focus merely shifts to timing and not nutritional value. Strive for a balanced intake of macronutrients and micronutrients through a varied and colorful diet guaranteeing a wide range of nutritional benefits. Regularly utilizing a food tracker or consulting a dietitian can ensure you're eating a balanced diet.

8.4. Overcoming Social Pressures

Mealtimes often are a social activity, and your new eating regimen may disrupt this, causing isolation or misunderstanding. To combat this, communication is instrumental. Informing those around you about your dietary approach enables them to support you. Also, strive to retain social interactions around meals—you can participate by enjoying a calorie-free drink while others eat, or schedule social engagements around your feeding window.

8.5. Navigating the Intermittent Fasting Dips

Even with the best preparation and tactics, intermittent fasting will have peaks and troughs. There will be days when your hunger and cravings are particularly intense, contributing to the challenge. Patience and flexibility are key during these times. A rough day or week doesn't mean failure but a part of the process. If required, adjust your fasting period to a time that suits you better.

Assessing beforehand potential obstacles and developing techniques to tackle them immensely helps in this journey. Remember, a successful transition to intermittent fasting is less about perfect execution and more about persistence and adaptability. Making incremental adjustments while remembering the bigger picture—the improved health outcomes and vitality—is crucial to overcoming the common challenges of intermittent fasting.

Chapter 9. Incorporating Intermittent Fasting into Your Lifestyle

The decision to incorporate intermittent fasting into your lifestyle is a step towards a healthier, more balanced life. The intermittent fasting approach can seem a bit daunting at first, but with time, information, and practical guidance, you'll find it surprisingly easy to fit into your daily routine.

9.1. Understanding Intermittent Fasting

Before diving into the particulars of how to incorporate intermittent fasting, it's vital to understand what it truly is. Intermittent Fasting (IF) refers to a meal timing schedule that flips between voluntary fasting periods and designated eating windows. It's important to note here that IF is about 'when' you eat, not 'what' you eat. However, it must not be seen as an excuse to consume unhealthy food during your eating windows. Nourishing diet in combination with IF will maximize health benefits and achieve the best possible outcomes.

9.2. Choosing Your Fasting Protocol

Intermittent fasting comes with a host of methods, each with its unique fasting and eating periods. Some of the popular methods include:

- 16:8 Method: Involves a 16-hour fasting window and an 8-hour eating window.

- 5:2 Method: Incorporates two fasting days with a restriction of

500-600 calories, with five normal eating days.

- Eat-Stop-Eat: Encompasses a 24-hour fast once or twice a week.

- Alternate-Day Fasting: Involves fasting every other day.

The key lies in choosing a method that suits your lifestyle, health goals, and general comfort. Experiment with the various options and stick to the one that feels sustainable and beneficial over the long term.

9.3. Preparing for the Transition

The transition to intermittent fasting should ideally be gradual, giving your body time to adapt to the new eating schedule. Start by extending your overnight fast a few hours at a time. Increase your fasting window gradually until you reach your desired fasting period. During your eating windows, prioritize foods high in proteins, healthy fats, and fiber to keep you feeling fuller for longer and maintain your energy levels.

9.4. Overcoming Common Challenges

During the initial stages, you may encounter some challenges like hunger pangs, fatigue, or lightheadedness as your body adjusts to the new routine. Staying hydrated during your fasting window can often help with hunger and fatigue. Black coffee, tea, and other non-caloric beverages are also beneficial to keep feeling full and energized. If the side effects continue or become severe, consult with a healthcare provider.

9.5. Combining IF with Exercise

Exercise and fasting are not mutually exclusive; in fact, they can compliment each other quite well. Exercising in a fasted state can help maximize fat burning. To ensure adequate energy during workouts, try to schedule your workouts towards the end of your fasting period, right before your first meal.

9.6. Monitor Your Progress

Keeping a food and fasting diary can be instrumental in tracking your development, identifying patterns, and making necessary adjustments. Record the duration of your fasts, your meals, your feelings, and any body changes. This documented journey will hold invaluable insights to maximize the health benefits of intermittent fasting.

9.7. Listening to Your Body

Finally, it's crucial to listen to your body. As you progress, adjustments to your eating window, fasting period, or meal choices could be required. If intermittent fasting feels too restrictive or starts interfering with your sleep, your mood, or your ability to concentrate, it may not be the right fit for you. Make sure that any diet protocol you subscribe to contributes positively towards your overall life quality.

While the thought of incorporating changes into your existing lifestyle might be overwhelming at first, the initial discomfort and adjustments pave way for a multitude of long-term health benefits. As intermittent fasting grows to become a part of your daily routine, you'll inevitably witness a remarkable transformation in your health, waistline, and overall well-being. Remember, good health is a journey—not a destination—and every positive choice brings you one step closer to your goals.

Chapter 10. Real-life Success Stories of Intermittent Fasting

Success is the best motivator and real-life stories act as compelling testimonials of the effectiveness of intermittent fasting. As a part of this guide, we are going to dive into the inspiring stories of people who have witnessed striking transformations in their health and body, thanks to the power of intermittent fasting.

10.1. The Story of Emily: Turning the Tides with Intermittent Fasting

Emily, a 38-year-old mother of two, had slowly gained weight after her pregnancies. Increasing caregiving duties led Emily to slip into a spiral of unhealthy eating habits and a sedentary lifestyle. Over time, she watched her energy levels deplete and her waistline increase. One day, she decided that change was crucial.

Emily stumbled upon the concept of intermittent fasting during her quest to regain control of her health. She started with the 16:8 fasting regime, meaning she ate within an 8-hour window and fasted for 16 hours. Initially, it was a struggle as her body was accustomed to regular meals interspersed with uncontrolled snacking. Despite the initial resistance, Emily continued with her plan.

A month into her new lifestyle regime, Emily started noticing some key changes. She felt more energized, alert, and her clothes fit better. Her food cravings had notably decreased, and her portion control improved. By the sixth month, she had dropped two clothes sizes, boasting an impressive reduction in waist circumference.

Emily's story proves that with the right determination and consistency, intermittent fasting can prompt beneficial changes to our health and physique.

10.2. The Journey of Martin: From Sedentary to Spirited

Martin, at the age of 45, was leading an exceptionally sedentary lifestyle due to his desk job. His increasing weight exacerbated pre-existing health conditions, threatening his overall well-being. Martin's doctor warned him about the dangers of his deteriorating health condition and urged him to make lifestyle changes.

Martin started researching different dietary protocols and soon came upon intermittent fasting. He was attracted by its simplicity and the freedom it offered from strict meal planning. Starting with a 16:8 fasting routine, Martin committed to this new lifestyle change.

He faced difficulties at first, but gradually his body adjusted to the new eating schedule. Martin reported feeling lighter and more energetic within the first few weeks. In combination with moderate exercise, he also observed a significant change in his body composition and mental clarity. It wasn't long before he had lost several pounds, managed to keep them off, and significantly improved his health markers.

Martin's story illustrates how intermittent fasting can revive one's health and vigor, proving to be a powerful tool in the journey towards a healthier lifestyle.

10.3. Lisa's Transformation: Defying Age with Intermittent Fasting

Lisa, a 56-year-old woman, had always struggled with yo-yo dieting.

Over the decades, her weight fluctuated wildly, leading to frustration and a sense of defeat. As she aged, she began to fear the impact of her inconsistent dietary habits on her overall health and longevity.

Lisa discovered intermittent fasting while browsing the internet for weight management tips. Intrigued, she decided to give the 5:2 intermittent fasting regime a try, where she ate normally for five days of the week and restricted her calories to 500-600 on two non-consecutive days.

Adjusting to the 5:2 regimen was challenging at first, but Lisa persevered. After several weeks, she noticed that she had more energy, her skin looked healthier, and she began losing weight at a steady pace. Beyond just the weight loss, Lisa found herself feeling more confident and in control of her nutrition and health. Upon her most recent medical check-up, Lisa was delighted to discover that her blood pressure, cholesterol and blood sugar levels had all improved.

Lisa's journey constitutes a powerful testament that it's never too late to start intermittent fasting and highlights the pronounced changes this practice brings about – not just in physique, but overall well-being and self-esteem.

Through Emily, Martin, and Lisa's stories, we've seen how incremental lifestyle changes, like adopting intermittent fasting, induced significant health and body transformations. Remember, every piece of evidence, whether scientific or anecdotal, brings us another step closer to understanding the true impact of intermittent fasting on our health.

Chapter 11. The Future of Intermittent Fasting: What Research Tells Us

Despite the burgeoning intrigue around intermittent fasting (IF), some are concerned about its long-term impacts and potential hurdles in further investigations. The current landscape of proliferative scientific research into IF holds promising prospects, albeit embedded within its limitations and controversies. Therefore, a comprehensive understanding of scientific implications is vital to envision the future of IF.

11.1. Current Research on Intermittent Fasting

Intermittent fasting has become a focal point of dietary research due to its ability to promote weight loss and improve metabolic health. Numerous animal and human studies have been conducted to understand its physiological effects and potential health benefits.

One prominent sphere of intermittent fasting revolves around its impact on weight loss and metabolism. Various studies have demonstrated its role in promoting weight loss, improving metabolic health, and reducing the risk of chronic diseases such as diabetes, heart diseases, and cancer. In a 2019 study published in the "New England Journal of Medicine," a team of researchers outlined the numerous benefits of intermittent fasting, including improved stress resistance, increased lifespan, and enhanced cognitive health.

However, research indicates that these benefits extend beyond weight-loss and metabolic optimization. Evidence from animal studies demonstrates that intermittent fasting can enhance cognitive function and resistance to stress and disease. A study published in "Cell Metabolism" in 2018 reported improved memory and learning among rats that followed an intermittent fasting diet.

11.2. Limitations and Controversies in Current Research

While the body of animal-based research on intermittent fasting is substantial, human pieces of evidence are scattered and, in some respects, contradictory. The limitations of current research lie fundamentally in its relatively short-term span and lack of consistency in defining fasting protocols leading to discrepancies.

One controversy revolves around the differential impact of intermittent fasting on men and women. A 2017 study published in "JAMA Internal Medicine" conducted on 100 individuals over a year, concluded that IF did not outperform other weight-loss strategies. Furthermore, some studies indicate that intermittent fasting could potentially lead to menstrual irregularities and fertility problems among women.

11.3. The Path to Future Research

Given the promising yet convoluted picture of IF, future research needs extensive, robust, and long-term human trials to unravel the web of its effects. It would involve identifying optimal fasting regimens considering factors such as age, sex, current health status, and genetic predispositions.

Research could further focus on nuances of intermittent fasting, like the influence of the timing of fasting–eating windows on health and weight outcomes. Observational studies, following people who naturally follow IF, could also provide insightful data, particularly about its long-term effects.

11.4. The Intersection of Interpersonal Differences and Intermittent Fasting

In addition to physiological health, the psychosocial aspects of intermittent fasting are also emerging as research interests. Sophisticated investigations could be made on how individual differences impact the response to IF, and vice versa. Looking at how personality, mood, behavior, culture, and social norms interact with the dietary practice can yield a more comprehensive understanding of its long-term viability.

Furthermore, future research should include widespread populations, diverse in age, race, and health status, to discover how IF impacts different demographics and whether it can be universally recommended. The advent of personalized medicine also signals the need for IF regimes tailored for individuals based on their unique physiology and lifestyle.

11.5. Technological Advancements and the Future of Intermittent Fasting

Of note is the potential role of technology in future intermittent fasting studies and dissemination. Wearable technology can aid in conducting large-scale, real-time, and accurate monitoring of individual's fasting regimens and body responses. Additionally, AI models could predict optimal intermittent fasting protocols for individuals based on a host of information like genetic markers, lifestyle habits, and current health status.

11.6. The Future Landscape of Intermittent Fasting

Given the complexity of the human body and the myriad of factors influencing health outcomes, the path towards fully understanding intermittent fasting is challenging but intriguing. While current research has started to unravel its tremendous potential, it is just the tip of the iceberg.

The future of intermittent fasting research, poignant with technological advancements, individualized approaches, and a holistic understanding of health, holds the promise of unfolding the full spectrum of its potential impact. However, only with rigorous, robust, and comprehensive scientific research can we anticipate fully utilizing IF as an effective tool for health optimization and disease prevention.

Remember, knowledge is fluid and dynamic; hence, our understanding of intermittent fasting's health effects will evolve as more research is being conducted. Keep abreast of the latest research and ensure to consult with healthcare professionals before embarking on any lifestyle shifts, including intermittent fasting.